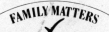

COMMON AILMENTS CURED NATURALLY

GW00601075

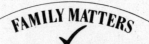

COMMON AILMENTS CURED NATURALLY

CAROLINE WHEATER

WARD LOCK

First published in 1990 by Ward Lock
Artillery House, Artillery Row, London SW1P 1RT, England

A Cassell imprint

© Ward Lock Limited 1990

British Library Cataloguing in Publication Data
Wheater, Caroline
  Common ailments cured naturally.
  1. Medicine. Natural remedies
  I. Title II. Series
  615.5'35

  ISBN 0–7063–6895–9

Printed and bound in Great Britain by William Collins & Sons, Glasgow

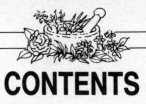

CONTENTS

INTRODUCTION

Good health is important to us all: it gives us energy to do things and enables us to have long and happy lives. Some bouts of ill health are unavoidable – an accident say, or a tropical disease – but in general the type of health problems the majority of us suffer from are minor but aggravating. But if left to fester they can herald a more serious problem in later life, such as heart disease or obesity.

Many practitioners of complementary health therapies believe that certain degenerative diseases such as multiple sclerosis and cancer may have a causal link to our lifestyles, diet and attention to health. It appears that how you treat your body, from childhood to old age can make a difference to your health. For this reason it is important to treat your body with respect.

The best way to maintain your health is with prevention in mind, and by taking into account your whole body. Drugs obtained from your doctor may just suppress the problem rather than effect a complete cure. Holistic health care is about returning your body to its normal balance, stimulating a strong immune system.

The therapies mentioned in this book all treat the person as a whole and not just the individual parts that sometimes become unwell. The root cause of a problem is often not visible, but hidden elsewhere in the body or to be found in the lifestyle or diet of a patient.

When giving a diagnosis, holistic therapists take into account your diet, your lifestyle, other health problems, hereditary links, your emotions, fears and character. This detailed survey gives them a much clearer picture of why a person is suffering from a certain problem. An insomniac may need to learn how to relax, whilst a person suffering from continuous colds, sore throats and flu may have a low immunity which needs boosting.

The remedies used in this book are all based on a holistic attitude to health and an idea that you don't have to rely on drugs to provide a solution to a problem. There are simple ways of giving your body a helping hand, through a wholesome diet, extra supplementation when needed, homoeopathic remedies, herbal medicine and aromatherapy oils.

We do stress, however, that serious complaints and problems that do not clear up quickly should always be taken to a qualified medical doctor for diagnosis. It is also wise to inform him or her of any other therapies you may be using, such as herbal infusions, supplements and homoeopathy. Never stop taking a prescribed drug without telling your GP.

It is also important to remember that many of these treatments are to be used now and again, not all the time. For example, for any long-term homoeopathic treatment you should be under the supervision of a qualified homoeopath, similarly with herbal medicine. The suggestions given in this book are for adults, and if treating a child you should seek professional advice.

If you would like to see a complementary therapist, contact the associations listed at the end of each section. They will be able to provide you with the name and address of a fully qualified therapist in your area. As well as specific suppliers given in this book, many wholefoods, supplements and remedies are available from health food stores nationwide.

THE IMPORTANCE OF DIET

The old adage 'we are what we eat' is the key to healthy living. A body needs a mixture of nutritious foods to be at its best. Foods contain important vitamins and minerals which we can't manufacture in our bodies, and which we need to function in top gear. They also provide energy in the form of fat, protein, and carbohydrates.

The average British diet contains far too many fatty foods such as butter, cream, fried food and fatty meat, and far too many refined, sugary carbohydrates such as cakes, biscuits, chocolate and processed foods. It doesn't contain enough unrefined carbohydrates such as cereals, seeds, pulses, potatoes, wholemeal bread and pasta, which also provide valuable fibre, or enough fruit and vegetables.

A healthy wholefood diet should give you much more energy and more resistance to infections, and as long as you get plenty of exercise and are not too highly stressed, you should have a much higher standard of health than if you were eating a bad refined and processed diet. Food near to its natural state also contains essential nutrients in a highly digestible form.

Of course, everyone slips up now and again, and that's permissible, as long as the majority of the food you eat is 'real food'. Follow the simple rule of not eating anything to excess; make sure that every day you eat fresh vegetables and fruit, a source of protein and unrefined carbohydrate with fibre. Try to reduce your intake of red meat, and concentrate instead on eating more fish, white meat and vegetarian forms of protein.

WHY DO WE NEED SUPPLEMENTS?

Sometimes we don't have enough time to eat properly, or the food that we do eat is not high enough in nutrients. This is where food supplements, such as vitamins and minerals come in handy. They are essential to health and can also give the body a much-needed boost when under the weather. Ideally, you should be taking a high quality multi-vitamin and mineral supplement every day.

When choosing your supplement always opt for the 'chelated' version if there is one. (This means that the substance has already been changed into its digestible form during manufacture and that, as a result, your body will absorb much more of it.) Also look for tablets or capsules that work on a time-release basis. This means that once inside your digestive system, they will release their contents slowly and more effectively.

HOW TO FIND OUT MORE ABOUT DIET AND SUPPLEMENTS

A Qualified Naturopath:

Contact the British Naturopathic and Osteopathic Association, 6 Netherhall Gardens, London NW3 5RR, telephone 01–435 8728.

Quality Supplements:

Nature's Best, 1 Lambert's Road, Tunbridge Wells, Kent TN2 3EQ, telephone 0892 34143.

Cantassium, 225 Putney Bridge Road, London SW15 2PY, telephone 01–874 1130.

G.R. Lane, Sisson Road, Gloucester, GL1 3QB, telephone 0452 24012.

Body Active, The London Pavilion, 1 Piccadilly Circus, London W1V 9LA, telephone 01–494 0841.

G & G Food Supplies, 175 London Road, East Grinstead, West Sussex, RH19 1YY, telephone 0342 312811.

THE BENEFITS
OF HOMOEOPATHY

Homoeopathy is now practised by 600 orthodox medical doctors in Britain and there are six NHS homoeopathic hospitals. It can no longer be described as a fringe medicine by its critics. Homoeopathic remedies have helped many people who dislike the side-effects of modern drugs or for whom orthodox treatment has had little success. Many GPs now realize that homoeopathic remedies can and do work, given the chance.

Homoeopathy is based on a theory developed by Dr. Samuel Hahnemann in the early part of the last century. His idea was that to make people better, you treated them with substances that, when given to a healthy person, mimicked the symptoms of the patient's infection. Hence the saying 'treating like with like'. Modern medicine rests on the concept that illness is treated with opposite substances that block or attack the infection.

Modern homoeopathic remedies are diluted to such a point that they actually contain only a few or no molecules of the original substance. When Hahnemann began to dilute his remedies, he found that they were more effective and faster working than the undiluted ones.

So where's the logic behind this? Homoeopaths

believe that through the process of dilution, the original healing substance leaves a blueprint on the remaining molecules of the substance used to dilute (either lactose or alcohol). This blueprint collects energy and the more it is diluted the more energy there is.

A remedy such as Arnica 6c has been diluted a hundredfold, six times. Arnica 30c will have been diluted a hundredfold, 30 times and in homoeopathic terms is stronger than Arnica 6c. The more the substance is diluted, the more healing energy is packed into the molecules.

The remedies, and there are more than 2,000 of them, usually take the form of tiny pills (pilules), which are tasteless, or liquid solutions, known as Mother Tinctures. Some of them also come in the form of a cream or ointment. They are derived from plant, animal and chemical origins and all have Latin names, which can be rather off-putting! Homoeopathic remedies should be kept somewhere cool and dark, in sealed containers.

FIRST AID BOX

★ *Pilules:*	Aconite; Apis; Arnica; Arsen Alb; Belladonna; Bryonia; Carbo Veg; Chamomilla; Hepar Sulph; Nux Vomica; Pulsatilla; Sulphur.
★ *Mother Tinctures:*	Calendula, Euphrasia, Hypericum, Pyrethrum.
★ *Salves:*	Arnica; Calendula; Hypericum.

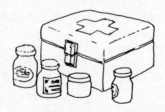

HOW TO FIND OUT MORE ABOUT HOMOEOPATHY

A Qualified Homoeopath:

Contact The British Homoeopathic Association, 27a Devonshire Street, London WC1N 1RJ, telephone 01–935 2163, or The Society of Homoeopaths, 47 Canada Grove, Bognor Regis, West Sussex, PO21 1DW, telephone 0243 860678.

Quality Homoeopathic Remedies:

Ainsworths, 38 New Cavendish Street, London, W1M 7LH, telephone 01–935 5330.

Buxton and Grant, 176 Whiteladies Road, Bristol, BS8 2XU, telephone 0272 735025.

Galen Pharmacy, 1 South Terrace, South Street, Dorchester, Dorset, DT1 1DE, telephone 0305 63996.

Goulds, 14 Crowndale Road, London NW1 1TT, telephone 01–388 4752.

Nelson's Pharmacies Ltd, 73 Duke Street, London W1M 6BY, telephone 01–629 3118.

Weleda, Heanor Road, Ilkeston, Derbyshire, DE7 8DR, telephone 0602 303151.

HERBAL MEDICINE

Modern herbal medicine has its roots far back in history. Until the seventeenth century, it was the only kind of medicine available. The physics of the time were well trained in the uses of many different types of herb and would prescribe them accordingly for every kind of illness.

Herbal medicine has thousands of years of research and experience to offer – herbs were used by many ancient civilizations too.

Herbal medicines are taken as teas, tinctures, inhalations and salves and help return an unhealthy body to a state of 'homoeostasis' or balance. They don't actually 'cure' in the sense of the word, but they stimulate the body to cure itself.

Taken properly, herbs are safe, but you should bear in mind that they are also powerful substances that can cause ill-effects if taken in too strong a dose. It is best to consult a medical herbalist if you wish to treat anything serious or over a long time-span.

Dried herbs are normally used to make teas (recommended in this book), and the ratio is one teaspoon to a cupful, or 25 g (1 oz) to a 600 ml (one pint), of boiling water. If you can obtain fresh herbs, you will need to use three times as much as the dried variety (i.e. three teaspoons and 75 g (3 oz). Leaves, stems and flowers are infused, usually in a teapot, with hot water; but bark and tougher roots are used in a 'decoction' – where they are simmered in boiling water for a few minutes to release the goodness. Always strain the liquid before drinking.

If herbal teas taste too bitter to drink, add a little liquorice or honey. Many herbs can be used in cooking to impart healthy benefits through food – use as often as possible.

FIRST AID BOX

★ **Dried herbs:** Chamomile; Cloves; Comfrey; Cramp Bark; Elderflower; Eyebright; Ginger; Hyssop; Liquorice; Nettles; Marigold; Meadowsweet; Pennyroyal; Rosemary; Sage; Scullcap; Slippery Elm; Thyme.

★ **Creams/oils/ lotions:** Aloe gel; Marigold cream; oil of St. John's Wort.

HOW TO FIND OUT MORE ABOUT HERBAL MEDICINE

A Qualified Medical Herbalist:

Contact the National Institute of Medical Herbalists, 41 Hatherley Road, Winchester, Hampshire, SO22 6RR, telephone 0962 68776, or the General Council and Register of Consultant Herbalists, Marlborough House, Swanpool, Falmouth, Cornwall, TR11 4HW, telephone 0326 317321.

Quality Herbs:

Baldwins, 171 Walworth Road, London SE17, telephone 01–701 4892 (mail order available).

Neal's Yard Remedies, 2 Neal's Yard, Covent Garden, London WC2, telephone 01–379 7222. Branches also in Oxford and Totnes (mail order available).

Culpeper Ltd, 21 Bruton Street, London SW1, telephone 01–629 4559 (mail order available).

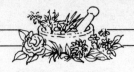

AROMATHERAPY

The healing art of aromatherapy is closely linked to herbalism, as it uses essential oils extracted from plants and flowers. Aromatherapy was so named by a French scientist named Gattefosse, early this century. One day while in his laboratory he burnt his hand, nearby lay a dish of lavender oil. He quickly put the burnt area into the dish, and was astonished to find how quickly the burn healed up.

When Gattefosse published his first book on the topic in 1928, he opened up a whole new field of interest, and from that point on, scientists, doctors and biochemists have continued to find out about the hidden qualities of plant oils. Of course, Gattefosse's discovery was not new: the Egyptians used essential oils for everything, including the process of mummifying bodies! It was also used by the Greeks and Romans.

Essential plant oils are extracted by distillation or effleurage (when the essence is absorbed by fat or vegetable oil and then separated). All the oils contain anti-microbial, antiseptic properties, and because they are collected in a very concentrated form are much more powerful than if, for instance, you were to rub a rose petal on your skin.

Essential oils can be extracted from flowers, bark, leaves, fruits and resins. Aromatherapists mix small amounts of the oils with a carrier oil (almond and soya oil are nice light oils to use), and then massage the liquid into the skin. Once on the skin, research has shown that it is absorbed into the blood stream, by penetrating the dermis (inner layer of the skin).

Essential oils can also be inhaled and added to your bath. Because of their concentrated strength they should not be taken internally, unless instructed by a qualified aromatherapist. Although quality essential oils are expensive, they are much more effective. Some oils on sale are low grade and made for the cosmetics industry – they are not suitable for health treatments. The fun thing about aromatherapy is that you can experiment for yourself, find out what smells you like, and adjust the recipes to fit. If you can, make sure that you buy organic oils.

A WORD OF WARNING

Certain oils can cause miscarriage in pregnant women. If pregnant, you should avoid oils extracted from spices, herbs and resins; but flower oils are generally fine. Use Frankincense, Jasmin Rose, Melissa Rose, Sweet French Marjoram, Mandoine, Ylang Ylang, Chamomile Flower, Orange Blossom, Petite Grain, Perma Rosa or Rosewood. If you are feeling sick, try Peppermint; if suffering from congestion try Honey Myrtle. At the end of the pregnancy use Rosemary or Lavender.

FIRST AID BOX

★ *Essential oils:*   Basil; Cajuput; Chamomile; Eucalyptus; Geranium; Ginger; Hyssop; Juniper; Lavender; Lemon; Marjoram; Myrrh; Peppermint; Pine; Rosemary; and Thyme.

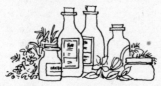

HOW TO FIND OUT MORE ABOUT AROMATHERAPY

A Qualified Aromatherapist:

Contact The Association of Tisserand Aromatherapists, PO Box 746, Brighton, East Sussex, BN1 3BN, or The Shirley Price Aromatherapy Group, Wesley House, Stockwell Head, Hinckley, Leicestershire, LE10 1RD, telephone 0455 615466 or The International Federation of Aromatherapists, 46 Dalkeith Road, London SE21 8LS, telephone 01-670 5011.

Quality Oils:

Shirley Price Oils, address as above.

Tisserand Oils, address as above.

Marguerite Maury Clinic, Park Lane Hotel, Piccadilly, London W1Y 8BX.

Neal's Yard Remedies, 2 Neal's Yard, Covent Garden, London WC2, telephone 01–379 7222.

Body Treats, 15 Approach Road, Raynes Park, London SW20 8BA, telephone 01–543 7633.

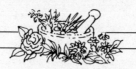

AN A TO Z OF AILMENTS AND TREATMENTS

ACNE

Acne is most common in teenagers and young adults for whom the problem is either hereditary or due to hormonal imbalance. In females acne can flare up before and during a period. Acne occurs because the skin's sebaceous glands produce too much grease and are infected by bacteria. This results in blackheads, lumpy spots and whiteheads. The biggest concentration of sebaceous glands is on the face, shoulders, chest and back and that's why spots always appear in these areas.

Some girls are prescribed the Contraceptive Pill to boost their level of female hormones and stop a hormonal imbalance. Many naturopaths believe that diet can help in ousting acne and that stress and emotional upset have an unhelpful effect on acne sufferers. Acne spots should never be picked, as scarring and further infection can result. Getting rid of acne is a very long term process so don't give up too soon – give any treatment at least three months to work.

Diet

★ *AVOID* chocolate, foods high in fat, sugary foods, tea and coffee.

★ **EAT MORE**   fresh fruit (citrus especially) and green leafy vegetables. Encourage good bowels by eating fibrous foods such as prunes, oats or bran, or take a spoonful of Castor oil – then the skin does not become overloaded with toxins.

Beneficial Supplements

Vitamin A (7500 IU daily)
Zinc (25 mg daily)
Evening Primrose oil (2 x 500 mg daily)

Homoeopathy

Chosen remedy to be taken over two weeks, three times daily.
Kali Bromatum 6c: for chronic acne, itchy
Sulphur 6c: chronic acne, chilly
Graphites 6c: infected, pus-filled spots
Hepar Sulph 6c: inflamed, boil-like spots
Calcarea Sulph 6c: pus-filled spots, heal slowly

Herbal Remedies

★ **Decoction:**   (for tea) dried Burdock root, Yellow Dock root and Sarsaparilla root. Add 1 oz (25 g) of the combination to a saucepan (not aluminium) of boiling water. Simmer with lid on for fifteen minutes. This will make three or four cups of tea. Strain and drink hot, one cupful three times daily.

★ **Compress:**   soak a piece of clean linen or gauze in a bowl of hot, infused Marigold or Witchhazel. To make infusion, pour boiling water over one heaped teaspoon of either herb and let stand for ten minutes. Place compress over affected area of skin, repeat a couple of times. Do this once a day.

Aromatherapy Oils

★ **Massage oil:** make a combination oil using five drops of Lavender, three drops of Cajuput, three drops of Chamomile and three drops of Juniper to 50 ml (2 fl oz) of Almond or Soya oil. Massage a little into affected skin once or twice daily.

★ **Bath oil:** add four drops of Lavender and four drops of Geranium to your bath.

ARTHRITIS AND RHEUMATISM

There are two types of arthritis: rheumatoid and osteo. Both conditions involve pain and restricted movement. Rheumatism is an umbrella term for any other aches and pains around the joints, often brought on by damp weather.

In rheumatoid arthritis, wrists and knuckles tend to become the most tender and inflamed parts of the body. Many doctors believe that it is caused by the immune system mistakenly attacking its own tissues. Women suffer more than men, but it can affect people of all ages.

Osteo-arthritis is when the cartilage linings around a joint degenerate, causing some pain and stiffness, but no inflammation. The most frequently affected areas are those joints which are heavily used, and often abused by bad posture, such as hips, knees and fingers. Osteo-arthritis is much more a disease of the elderly.

Diet

★ *AVOID*   refined foods such as white flour and rice, sugar, animal fats, salt and pepper.

★ *EAT PLENTY*   of raw fruit and vegetables, vegetable juices, wholegrain flour and rice, seaweed (like lava bread), pulses and seeds. Intersperse with fish, cheese, eggs and white meat for protein.

Beneficial Supplements

Kelp tablets (seaweed rich in minerals)
Cod Liver oil
Green-lipped mussel supplement
Selenium (50 mcg daily)
Vitamin C (1 g daily)
Vitamin B3 (50 mg daily)
Calcium Pantothenate (100 mg daily) may help

Homoeopathy

Take chosen remedy over two weeks three times daily

Osteoarthritis:
Rhus Tox 6c: for stiffness and aching, relief from heat
Bryonia 6c: symptoms aggravated by movement and heat, relief from cold
Calcarea Phos 6c: numbness, stiff, affected by weather

Rheumatoid Arthritis and Rheumatism:
Apis 6c: painful swelling
Belladonna 6c: heat makes it worse
Medorrhinum 6c: pain worse in mornings
Aconite 6c: sudden, searing pains
Pulsatilla 6c: pains move around body

Herbal Remedies

★ **Infusion:** (for tea) Bogbean, Meadowsweet and Ash. Add a heaped teaspoonful of this mixture to a teapot and cover with a cupful of boiling water. Infuse for ten minutes then drink. Take once or twice daily.

★ **Tincture:** Rub a combination of Cayenne and Glycerine tinctures on to the affected area. Or use Oil of St John's Wort.

Aromatherapy Oils

★ **Massage oil:** make a combination oil using five drops of Thyme, five drops of Rosemary and five drops of Juniper to 50 ml (2 fl oz) Almond or Soya oil. Rub into painful areas.

★ **Bath soak:** add four drops of Thyme and four drops of Lemon to a warm bath and soak.

ASTHMA

Asthma is caused by the constriction of the tiny air tubes inside the lungs. These 'bronchi' become swollen and congested, usually due to an allergic reaction to substances such as dust, cat fur, pollens or smoke.

The constriction of the bronchi provokes breathlessness and the production of thick mucus which gives further discomfort. The classic characteristic of an asthma attack is that the patient wheezes as they breathe out. They can also undergo violent coughing as the lungs attempt to expel mucus.

An attack can be made worse by emotional stress or

panic. The conventional treatment of asthma is normally with steroids, adrenalin type drugs and sometimes, in very severe cases, with hydro-cortisone. Sufferers may grow out of attacks in adult life.

Diet

| ★ *AVOID* | dairy products which are mucus forming – yogurt is the exception to the rule as it is thought to guard against allergic reaction. Also avoid processed foods, tea, coffee and excessive amounts of alcohol. |
| ★ *EAT* | a high fibre diet with plenty of fresh fruit and vegetables, (garlic is very useful). Change to herb teas, vegetable and fruit juices. Drink plenty at the beginning of an attack to avoid dehydration. |

Beneficial Supplements

Multi-vitamin and mineral capsules
Vitamin B Complex (30 mg daily)
Vitamin B6 (50 mg twice daily)
Vitamin C (1 g daily)

Homoeopathy

Chosen remedy to be taken every half hour, up to ten times per attack.
Pulsatilla 6c: accumulation of phlegm in chest
Arsenicum 6c: restlessness and agitation
Cuprum 6c: for violent spasms
Kali Carb 6c: chilly, early morning attack
Antimonium Tart 6c: fatigue, pallor, wheezing, coldness

Herbal Remedies

★ *Infusion:* (for tea) Thyme or Red Clover. Add one heaped teaspoon of either dried herb to a teapot, cover with a cupful of boiling water, infuse for ten minutes then drink. Drink one cup three times daily during an attack.

Aromatherapy Oils

★ *Massage oil:* combine two drops of Eucalyptus and one drop of Cajuput to an eggcupful of Almond or Soya oil. Rub into chest.

★ *Inhalation:* add two drops of Pine and two drops of Eucalyptus to a bowl of boiling water. Place towel over head and inhale.

ATHLETE'S FOOT

A condition in which the skin becomes itchy and flakes off between the toes or on the soles of the feet, athlete's foot is a form of ringworm, a microscopic fungus. The infected area often forms a circular patch that radiates outwards, hence the name ringworm.

Athlete's foot thrives in warm, moist atmospheres – a sweaty foot inside an enclosed sock and shoe is the ideal environment. It is easily passed on to others, so public swimming is not advised. The condition is usually quite easy to heal, although it can linger.

Diet

The growth of fungus upsets the acid/alkaline balance of the foot which becomes too alkaline. Plenty of fruit and vegetables should be consumed to redress the balance towards acidity.

★ **AVOID**   processed foods, animal fat and sugar, salt and spices. Instead of meat, eat cheese, nuts and pulses for protein intake.

Beneficial Supplements

Vitamin A (up to 7500 IU daily)
Vitamin B6 (up to 25 mg daily)
Vitamin B Complex (up to 100 mg daily)

Homoeopathy

Treatment is not direct, but incorporates the whole body – see a homoeopath.

Herbal Remedies

★ **Tincture:**   Marigold tincture should be applied regularly to the affected foot.

★ **Powder:**   dust feet with Arrowroot powder to prevent further sweating and itching.

Aromatherapy Oils

★ **Massage oil:** add three drops of Marigold to an eggcupful of Almond or Soya oil, massage on to feet.

BACKACHE

One of the most common reasons for absenteeism, backache can afflict the young and the old alike. Many of the muscular twinges and pains are caused by bad posture and overstraining, putting the ligaments, tendons and bones out of balance. Specific causes include slipped discs, entrapment of the sciatic nerve and cracked vertebrae.

Back pain can be caused by a misaligned pelvis, hips

or even feet. Improving posture through a process such as the Alexander Technique, or consulting an osteopath or chiropractor to manipulate and massage the affected areas may prove extremely beneficial. Otherwise backache and muscle strain must heal through rest.

Diet

★ *AVOID*   drinking tea and coffee. Instead try diluted fruit juices, lemon and water and herb teas.

Stick to a basic wholefood diet with PLENTY of fruit and vegetables, eat fish, cheese, lean meat and pulses for protein.

Beneficial Supplements

Vitamin E (up to 100 IU daily)
Vitamin C (300 mg daily)

Homoeopathy

Take your chosen remedy three times daily over two weeks.
Natrum Mur 6c: severe backache
Arnica 6c: backache due to stress
Rhus Tox 6c: for backache that responds to heat and movement
Bryonia 6c: acts on aching joints, ie. hips
Nux Vomica 6c: dull pain, could be linked with constipation

Herbal Remedies

★ *Infusion:*   (for bath) make an infusion of fresh nettles by adding 100 g (4 oz) of the herb to a bowl of boiling water. Infuse for ten minutes then add strained liquid to a warm bath.

★ **Infusion:** (for tea) add one heaped teaspoon of a mixture of dried Juniper, Horsetail and Buchu to a teapot, cover with a cupful of boiling water. Infuse for ten minutes then drink. Take one to two cups daily during period of pain.

Aromatherapy Oils

★ **Massage oil:** add five drops of Rosemary, four drops of Thyme, three drops of Nutmeg and three drops of Origanum to 50 ml (2 fl oz) of Almond or Soya oil. Massage a little into the back daily.

BAD BREATH

Bad breath can be caused by a number of things, including indigestion, illness, lack of food, dental decay or gum disease. Breath can be sweetened or you can deal with the root of the problem. If the stomach is not secreting enough hydrochloric acid, bacteria may flourish causing foul smelling breath – this should be diagnosed by a doctor.

Diet

★ **AVOID** foods that you know give you indigestion. Excessive intake of carbohydrates can also result in fermentation of the stomach so – AVOID cakes, sweets, chocolates and canned soft drinks.

★ **EAT** less red meat, more fruit and vegetables, particularly raw carrots, celery, parsley and anything crunchy and fresh.

★ **EAT PLENTY**   of fibre to keep the digestive system in good working order.

Beneficial Supplements

Antacids such as liver salts and bicarbonate of soda to settle the stomach (one teaspoon every couple of hours mixed with water).

Hydrochloric Acid tablets (only if you are suffering from fermentation of the stomach and on the advice of your GP).

Homoeopathy

Take chosen remedy three times daily for a week.
Nux Vomica 6c: if the problem is a result of stomach upset
Carbo Veg 6c: tooth and gum decay
Spigelia 6c: tongue unhealthily coated with a yellow or white layer
Mercurius 6c: offensive breath and perspiration, tooth decay, yellow tongue

Herbal Remedies

★ **Infusion:**   (for mouthwash) Dill and Fennel. Add one heaped teaspoon of the dried herbs, mixed, to a teapot. Cover with one cupful of boiling water. Infuse for ten minutes; when cool enough use infusion as a mouthwash and gargle.

Aromatherapy Oils

★ **Mouthwash:**   choose from Myrrh, Nutmeg, Rosemary and Peppermint. Add one drop of the chosen oil to a cup of warm water and gargle, then spit out.

BODY ODOUR

Commonly termed BO, this can be an extremely embarrassing problem affecting teenagers upwards, and is caused by over-active sweat glands. Often it is simply due to bad hygiene, but it can also be linked with your state of health. Diabetics, for example, sweat more profusely than others and may have difficulty controlling body odour.

The condition can also be aggravated by eating particularly spicy or pungent food such as curries and garlic. As the skin is a major organ for expelling toxins, much of the odour seeps through the pores, giving that post-garlic smell!

Diet

★ *EAT PLENTY* of foods rich in zinc, magnesium and Vitamin B6. Zinc-rich foods are red meat, egg yolks, oats, peanuts, split peas, potatoes and carrots. Magnesium-rich foods are nuts, shrimps, soya beans and green leafy vegetables. Foods rich in Vitamin B6 are meat, fish, nuts, seeds and wholegrain cereals.

Beneficial Supplements

Zinc (20 mg daily)
Magnesium (200 mg daily)
Vitamin B6 (25 mg daily)
Para-aminobenzoic acid (100 mg daily)

Homoeopathy

Take chosen remedy three times daily for a week.
Mercurius 6c: extreme sweating, nasty odour, could be due to illness
Nux Vomica 6c: extreme sweating through exertion
Bryonia 6c: sour smell

Herbal Remedies

★ *Powder:*   dust armpits with Arrowroot powder to help keep dry.

Aromatherapy Oils

★ *Massage oil:*   combine two drops of Bergamot and one drop of Cypress to an eggcupful of Almond or Soya oil. Massage into parts of body most affected.

BRONCHITIS

Fatigue, fever and a congested cough are all associated with bronchitis. It is an infection that inflames the tiny air passages in the lungs known as bronchi. The inflammation encourages the production of extra mucus which is coughed up. A dry cough often lingers long after the infection has gone.

For a quick recovery, the patient should be kept away from cold air, smoke and exertion. In some cases, the infection can be very severe – particularly in smokers – and can cause death. This form of infection is termed chronic bronchitis and the patient suffers from symptoms on a long-term basis. If this happens the tissues of the lungs are damaged and and not enough oxygen is transported into the blood stream.

Diet

★ *AVOID*   fatty foods, dairy produce and eggs which are mucus forming.

★ *EAT PLENTY*   of fruit and vegetables, homemade soups, wholemeal bread and pulses which are full of protein. Drink at least 1.75 litres (3 pints) of liquid a day, but NOT tea or coffee. Change to drinking herb teas (Rosehip tea especially as it is full of Vitamin C), fruit juices and mineral water.

| Beneficial Supplements |

Vitamin C (1 g daily)
Zinc in lozenge or tablet form (up to 25 mg daily)

| Homoeopathy |

Take the remedy of your choice every two to three hours for two days.

Bryonia 30c: has a soothing effect on the lungs and throat, a dry cough and headache

Belladonna 30c: high temperature, severe headache, skin hot to the touch

Hepar Sulph 6c: harsh cough, chilliness

Kali Bich 6c: can't cough up stringy phlegm

Aconite 30c: dry, hacking cough, chilliness, temperature

| Herbal Remedies |

★ **Cough Medicine:** containing Marshmallow, St John's Wort or Coltsfoot is particularly effective as an expectorant and calming agent. Aniseed cough mixture is quite safe for children.

★ **Infusion:** (for tea) Lungwort, Hyssop and Self-heal. Add 1 oz (25 g) of the combined herbs to a teapot, cover with 600 ml (1 pint) boiling water. Infuse for ten minutes. Drink three cups daily.

| Aromatherapy Oils |

★ **Massage oil:** add four drops of Eucalyptus, three drops of Hyssop, four drops of Pine and four drops of Lavender to 50 ml (2 fl oz) of Almond or Soya oil. Rub on to chest.

★ *Inhalation:*   add three drops of Pine and three drops of Lavender to a bowl of hot water, cover head with towel and inhale for five minutes.

BURNS AND SCALDS

When the skin is burnt, plasma, the fluid part of the blood leaks out into the body tissue to form blisters and swelling. In serious burns, plasma is reduced so dramatically that the circulation of the blood can slow right down putting the patient into shock. A bad but small burn can be less dangerous than burns covering much of the body for this reason.

In minor burns, a general rule of thumb is to run the burnt skin under cold water to stop further damage. Heat continues to radiate out from a burn for several minutes after it has taken place. The application of cold water rapidly slows this process down.

Diet

★ *EAT PLENTY*   of foods containing Vitamins C and E to help heal the skin quickly. Include blackcurrants (if in season), green leafy vegetables, sprouting seeds, wholegrains, pulses and peanuts.

Homoeopathy

Take chosen remedy three times daily for a week.
Mercurius 6c: extreme sweating, nasty odour, could be due to illness
Nux Vomica 6c: extreme sweating through exertion
Bryonia 6c: sour smell

Herbal Remedies

★ *Powder:*   dust armpits with Arrowroot powder to help keep dry.

Aromatherapy Oils

★ ***Massage oil:*** combine two drops of Bergamot and one drop of Cypress to an eggcupful of Almond or Soya oil. Massage into parts of body most affected.

Beneficial Supplements

Cod Liver oil
Rosehip syrup
Vitamin C (up to 5 g daily for more serious burns – on advice of doctor)
Vitamin E capsules (400 IU daily during the time when the burn is at its worst) – it can also be applied as a cream

Homoeopathy

Arnica 30c: severe burns with shock, up to three doses every 15 minutes
Urtica 6c: blistering or swelling less severe, up to six doses every 15 minutes
Causticum 6c: for burns that remain inflamed and sore, three times daily for five days.
Hypericum cream: applied to the burn.

Herbal Remedies

★ ***Skin applications:*** Aloe gel is soothing and cooling. If you have an Aloe plant, gel fresh from a broken leaf can be used. Calendula (Marigold) cream applied locally to a burn speeds up healing.

Aromatherapy Oils

★ ***Undiluted oil:*** Lavender can be applied to a burn in small quantities and has remarkable healing effects. Geranium and Chamomile are also recommended.

COLD SORES (*Herpes Simplex*)

Cold sores usually affect the skin around the mouth and nose. More often than not the infection originates from childhood when the patient has come into contact with the Herpes Simplex virus. Once contracted, the virus digs itself into the nerve endings and remains there permanently. Cold sores look like large blisters and initially produce pus, they also form unsightly scabs when healing.

A group or a single coldsore can develop at any time, more frequently when the person's immune system is at a low ebb, due to stress or bad diet. Cold sores can also be provoked by exposure to sunshine. They take between a week and ten days to clear up.

Diet

Excess mucus does not help a coldsore sufferer, so when you feel a coldsore developing,

★ *AVOID*   mucus-forming foods such as dairy products.

★ *EAT PLENTY*   of raw or lightly cooked fruit and vegetables, nuts, seeds, pulses, wholemeal bread, lean meat, chicken or fish.

Beneficial Supplements

Lysine (an amino-acid, 250 mg daily as a preventive measure)
Vitamin C (1 g daily)
Vitamin B6 (50 mg daily)
Vitamin B5 (also known as pantothenic acid, up to 100 mg daily)

Homoeopathy

Chosen remedy to be taken three times daily over five days.

Pulsatilla 6c: good for catarrh sufferers
Natrum Mur 6c: ideal for blisters with fluid

Herbal Remedies

★ *Infusion:* (for tea) Echinacea and Cleavers. Combine equal measures of the two herbs, add one heaped teaspoon to a teapot, cover with a cupful of boiling water, leave to infuse for ten minutes, then drink. Consume two cups of herb tea every day while the cold sore lasts.

★ *Skin application:* the juice of a lemon can have a healing effect on cold sores.

Aromatherapy Oils

★ *Direct application:* apply a drop of either Geranium or Lavender oil directly to the cold sore, three times daily.

COMMON COLD

This most frequent of infections still manages to baffle scientists and no company has yet come up with a cure for the cold. The only solution offered is to keep warm, drink plenty of liquids, eat wholesome food and take the odd aspirin.

The symptoms of a cold surface within forty-eight hours of being in contact with an infected person and include: blocked up nose, coughing, sore throat, headache and even a slight temperature. Most colds (there are over thirty different viruses) are gone within a few days, and should not be allowed to move down on to the chest.

Diet

★ *AVOID* refined, empty foods, that contain lots

of sugar but few nutrients such as buns, cakes and biscuits.

★ *EAT PLENTY* of raw garlic which has an excellent cleansing effect on the blood stream. Foods rich in Vitamin C will also help: citrus fruits, blackcurrants, peas, tomatoes, cherries, parsley, kale, broccoli, Brussels sprouts and cabbage.

Beneficial Supplements

Vitamin C (1 g daily)
Garlic perles (taken as directed on packet)

Homoeopathy

Chosen remedy to be taken every two hours up to four times a day.

Pulsatilla 6c: thick, yellow mucus, sense of taste and smell reduced

Allium Cepa 6c: watery mucus, sore lips and nose, sneezing

Arsenicum 6c: fatigue, sense of burning from watery mucus

Mercurius 6c: profuse sweating, sneezing, salivation, bad breath

Gelsemium 6c: flu–like symptoms, best tucked up in bed

Herbal Remedies

★ *Infusion:* (for tea) Elderflower and Peppermint. Combine equal parts and add one heaped teaspoon to a teapot. Add a cupful of boiling water and infuse for ten minutes, then drink. Taken three times daily, this tea will encourage sleep and sweating to help rid the body of the bug.

Aromatherapy Oils

★ *Inhalation:* add five drops of Eucalyptus to a bowl of boiling water, cover head with towel and inhale.

★ **Bath soak:**   add five drops of pine and three drops of thyme to a warm bath.

★ **Skin application:**   for sore nose and lips add three drops of Niaouli oil to an eggcupful of Almond or Soya oil and rub into surrounding skin.

CONJUNCTIVITIS

An inflamed, pink-looking eye is a sure sign of conjunctivitis. The eye will feel sore, discharge a yellowy substance and the lids will be a little swollen. True conjunctivitis is due to an infection, but the condition commonly known as 'pink eye' can also be caused by an allergy or a foreign body lodging itself in the eye, such as a piece of dust or grit. 'Pink eye' can also be a symptom of Vitamin B2 deficiency.

Diet

★ **EAT PLENTY**   of foods rich in Vitamin A, which is very beneficial for eye problems: fish liver oils, green and orange vegetables, orange fruits, dairy products and eggs.

Beneficial Supplements

Vitamin C (500 mg daily, if pinkness is caused by an allergy)
Vitamin B6 (50 mg daily)
Vitamin B2 (50 mg daily)
Vitamin A (5000 IU daily during infection)

Homoeopathy

Chosen remedy to be taken every two hours for up to ten doses a day.
Pulsatilla 6c: heavy yellow discharge, itching
Euphrasia 6c: swollen lids, watering
Aconite 6c: for sore, gritty feeling

Apis 6c: swollen eyelids and stinging sensation
Euphrasia mother tincture: ten drops to 300 ml (½ pint) water, add one teaspoon of salt and bathe eyes with solution

Herbal Remedies

★ ***Infusion:*** (for eyewash) Eyebright. Add 25 g (1 oz) of the dried herb to 600 ml (1 pint) of boiling water, infuse and strain. Wash eye in the cooled liquid twice daily, or soak a piece of linen or gauze in the infusion and use as a compress, placing over eye for ten minutes. Elderflower and Marigold can also be used in this way.

Aromatherapy Oils

★ ***Skin application:*** add one drop of Chamomile and one drop of Rose to an eggcupful of Almond oil, use to massage skin surrounding eye.

★ ***Eyewash:*** add one drop of Chamomile and one drop of Lemon to an eggcupful of warm water and bathe eye twice daily.

CONSTIPATION

When you have difficulty going to the toilet, your stools are uncomfortably hard or your movements are very irregular, it is likely that you are constipated. It is not true that you have to have a bowel movement every day otherwise you are constipated – we are all different. Some people have perfectly healthy bowels that work every two to three days.

The underlying root causes of constipation are often suppressed by the use of laxatives. Instead the sufferer should be looking at ways to correct this unhealthy situation permanently, which can be the cause of headaches, fatigue and bad breath. Today's highly processed diet does not help and a return to fresh and raw foods with plenty of roughage is essential, as is drinking lots of liquid to help the kidneys work to the maximum.

Sometimes constipation can be caused by obstructions in the bowel such as piles, benign growths or cancer, so an unusually protracted bout of constipation in adults should always be reported to the doctor. Some drugs for high blood pressure and depression can also cause constipation.

In general, constipation sufferers should review their diet, take more exercise and try to establish a regular pattern for bowel movements, i.e. after a meal.

Diet

★ *AVOID* processed foods, particularly those with empty calories such as cakes, buns, biscuits, crisps and some breakfast cereals.

★ *EAT PLENTY* of green leafy vegetables, nuts, beans, wholegrains, wholemeal bread and oats. Raw vegetables eaten in salads are particularly beneficial as they provide high amounts of roughage. Fruits such as dates, figs, raisins, prunes and apricots are well known for their laxative properties – but don't overdo it as they can give you stomach ache! Live yogurt helps to recolonize beneficial bacteria in the gut, if the sufferer has been on a course of antibiotics or is recovering from an upset stomach.

| Beneficial Supplements |

Agar Agar (sprinkle one teaspoon over food, daily)
Kelp tablets (six daily)
Vitamin B complex (up to 100 mg daily)

| Homoeopathy |

Chosen remedy to be taken every two hours up to ten times a day.
Bryonia 30c: absence of desire, hard dry stools
Nux Vomica 6c: for use after repeated phases of constipation
Natrum Mur 6c: bleeding, crumbly stool
Aesculus 6c: stabbing, spiky sensation in anus

| Herbal Remedies |

★ *Infusion:* (as laxative) Liquorice, Elderflower, Senna and Fennel Seed. Combine equal parts of the herbs, add one heaped teaspoon to a teapot, cover with a cupful of boiling water, infuse for ten minutes then drink. Take this infusion once daily, should a laxative be needed.

| Aromatherapy Oils |

★ *Massage oil:* add one drop Black Pepper, one drop Marjoram and one drop Rosemary to an eggcupful of Almond oil, rub into the stomach.

COUGHS

Coughs often accompany colds, sore throats and always bronchitis. It is an automatic reaction by the throat and lungs to expel an unwanted substance such as a crumb of food, dust or mucus. Coughs can be dry and extremely irritating or wet and very thick with mucus, causing an aching chest and severe fatigue.

Diet

★ *AVOID* dairy foods which are mucus forming (except yogurt).

★ *DRINK PLENTY* of liquids, particularly honey and lemon with hot water to lubricate throat.

★ *EAT PLENTY* of fresh fruit and vegetables to up your Vitamin C intake and boost your immune system.

Beneficial Supplements

Vitamin C (1 g daily)
Vitamin B Complex (up to 100 mg daily)

Homoeopathy

Chosen remedy to be taken over two days, maximum ten doses a day.
Bryonia 30c: dry cough, often with side pain and stitches
Ipecacuanha 6c: wheezy chest, wet cough
Pulsatilla 6c: thick phlegm, unhappy patient
Belladonna 30c: flushed, headache, dry cough
Rumex 6c: hacking, dry cough, set off by talking, cold air

Herbal Remedies

★ *Cough medicine:* buy a cough medicine that includes Coltsfoot, Marshmallow, Peppermint, Hyssop, Horehound or Liquorice.

★ *Infusion:* (for tea) combine Coltsfoot, Marshmallow and Liquorice in equal parts. Add 25 g (1 oz) of the mixture to 600 ml (1 pint) of boiling water and infuse for ten minutes. Drink one cup, then store the rest to be drunk throughout the day.

Aromatherapy Oils

★ *Massage oil:*   add two drops of Eucalyptus, one drop of Aniseed and two drops of Hyssop to an eggcupful of Almond oil. Massage into the chest.

★ *Inhalation:*   add five drops of Eucalyptus to a bowl of boiling water, cover head with towel and inhale for several minutes.

CRAMP

Cramps are involuntary muscle spasms which can be brought on by a number of causes including lack of salt, bad circulation and continuous use of certain muscles. Most common are night cramps in the legs, often after a day of strenuous exercise.

Cramp can also occur in the neck, the stomach, the feet and the hands. Once a cramp has developed, the only way to banish it is to stretch the muscle – painful but necessary. If the cramp stems from a circulation problem, you should try to take more exercise to stimulate the blood flow to all parts of the body. Massage should also be considered as a way of improving bad circulation.

Diet

★ *REDUCE*   intake of acid forming foods such as meat, chocolate, peanuts, cheese, eggs, butter, bread, fish, flour, grains, pasta and oatflakes.

★ INCREASE intake of alkali-forming foods like fruits, vegetables, milk, yogurt, fruit juice, honey, molasses and wine. Also increase salt if your diet is lacking, quite unlikely if you eat a lot of processed foods, but possible if you sweat a lot.

Beneficial Supplements

Multi-vitamin and Mineral supplement containing Vitamins A, C and D and minerals, Iron, Potassium, Magnesium and Calcium.

Vitamin B Complex (up to 100 mg daily)

or

Brewer's yeast tablets (six daily)

or

Molasses, which is a very good source of Vitamin B Complex and the above minerals – take two tablespoons daily.

Homoeopathy

Chosen remedy to be taken every five hours, up to six doses daily.

Cuprum 6c: cramp in leg muscles, toes and soles of feet

Kali Carb 6c: cramps in the middle of the night that awaken you

Arnica 30c: after unusual muscular exertion

Camphora 6c: cramp in calves

Herbal Remedies

★ Infusion: (for tea) Cramp Bark, Ginger and Scullcap. Combine equal parts and add one teaspoon of mixture to a teapot, cover with one cupful of boiling water and infuse for ten minutes, strain and drink before going to bed, or after exertion.

Aromatherapy Oils

★ *Massage oil:*   add five drops of Marjoram, five drops of Cinnamon and five drops of Thyme to 50 ml (2 fl oz) of Almond or Soya oil. Keep handy for rubbing into affected area, as these are all anti-spasmodic oils.

CUTS, BRUISES AND SPRAINS

Minor injuries to the skin and slightly more serious ones, such as sprains are something we all have to deal with, now and again. Cuts and bruises are seldom absent among young children and sprains can happen to anyone, given the wrong circumstances, from a fall or twisting your ankle, for example.

Sprains involve the tearing of ligaments close to the joint and therefore must be given time to recover properly, so that the ligaments knit together again. They are much more painful than a straightforward cut or bruise.

Diet

★ *INCREASE*   intake of foods rich in Vitamins A and E (the skin vitamins): Halibut Liver oil (best source), cheese, eggs and butter, green leafy vegetables, orange fruit, wheatgerm, wholegrain cereals.

Beneficial Supplements

Vitamin A (5000 IU daily)
Vitamin E (up to 100 IU daily)
Halibut Liver oil capsules (a natural supply of Vitamin A)

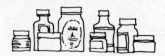

45

| Homoeopathy |

Chosen remedy to be taken three times daily for four days.

Arnica 30c: for shock, swelling and bruising
Arnica 30c, Rhus Tox 6c, Bellis 6c: for sprains
Calendula salve: for cuts and bruises

| Herbal Remedies |

★ *Ointment:*   for cuts use Comfrey, for bruises and sprains Calendula ointment.

★ *Infusions:*   (for bathing) Witchhazel and Thyme. Choose either herb and add one heaped teaspoon to a cupful of boiling water. Infuse for ten minutes, then apply to affected area, using a compress of linen or gauze.

| Aromatherapy Oils |

★ *Massage oil:*   for bruises and sprains add two drops of Myrrh, two drops of Lavender and two drops of Sage to an eggcupful of Almond oil. Massage on to affected area.

★ *Skin application:*   for cuts, dab a little of either Chamomile, Eucalyptus or Lavender diluted in Almond oil on to the wound.

CYSTITIS

Cystitis is a painful infection of the bladder caused by bacteria. The consequent inflammation can cause stomach and back ache, the passing of painful or burning urine sometimes containing blood or pus, and a feeling that you want to go to the toilet all the time.

Some sufferers also experience a fever with the

infection. Cystitis is not restricted to women, men can suffer too. Once a person has contracted it, cystitis appears to recur at intervals. One of the main origins of the bacteria is the anus, so take care to wipe your bottom from front to back to avoid spreading bacteria.

Diet

★ *AVOID*   highly spiced foods, foods with a high sugar content and alcohol which may irritate the bladder.

★ *DRINK PLENTY* of liquids, particularly diluted apple and grape juice, to help flush out the bacteria, when the inflammation first sets in.

★ *EAT*   a plain, but fresh, wholefood diet with plenty of fruit and vegetables.

Beneficial Supplements

Vitamin C (1 g daily)
Multi-vitamin and mineral supplement

Homoeopathy

Chosen remedy to be taken every half hour, up to ten doses per day.
Cantharis 30c: strong urge to urinate, stabbing pains in the abdomen
Apis 30c: bloody urine, feels hot, worse for heat
Hepar Sulph 6c: irritability and fatigue
Staphisagria 6c: after sex or use of a catheter, burning sensation

Herbal Remedies

★ *Infusion:* (for tea) Buchu, Couchgrass, Broom, Marshmallow. Combine in equal parts, add one heaped teaspoon of mixture to teapot cover with a cupful of boiling water. Leave to infuse for ten minutes, then drink. Marshmallow is particularly good for cystitis sufferers and can be drunk on its own as a tea.

Aromatherapy Oils

★ *Massage oil:* combine one drop of Juniper, one drop of Lavender, one drop of Cedarwood and two drops of Sandalwood to an eggcupful of Almond or Soya oil. Massage into the abdomen once a day during infection.

DANDRUFF

Dandruff is a result of over- or under-production of oil by the sebaceous glands in the scalp. Too little oil creates dry, white flaky bits of skin, too much oil produces yellow scales of skin. Dandruff can be linked to acne and can also be related to emotional health, illness, bad diet, strong shampoos and frequent hair washing in hot water. It often comes and goes, and scratching just makes it worse.

Diet

★ *AVOID* animal fats, processed carbohydrate foods, fried foods, spicy foods and alcohol, all of which can aggravate dandruff.

★ *DRINK PLENTY* of water, herb teas and fruit juices.

★ *INCREASE* intakes of wheatgerm, nuts and brewer's yeast.

Beneficial Supplements

Vitamin A (5000 IU daily)
Halibut Liver oil
Vitamin B6 (50 mg daily)
Vitamin B Complex (up to 100 mg daily)
Kelp tablets (six daily)

Homoeopathy

Chosen remedy to be taken four times daily over two weeks.

Sulphur 6c: with acne and itching scalp, hair washing makes it worse

Lycopodium 6c: a very dry skin

Oleander 6c: itching spots around forehead and at back of ears

Herbal Remedies

★ ***Infusion:*** (for tea) Burdock and Cleavers. Combine equal parts and add one heaped teaspoon to a teapot, cover with a cupful of boiling water, infuse for ten minutes, then drink.

★ ***Infusion:*** (for scalp treatment) Rosemary and Nettles. Combine equal parts of fresh herbs if possible, add 75 g (3 oz) to 600 ml (1 pint) boiling water, infuse for ten minutes then rub into clean scalp and leave on. Cider Vinegar and Lemon Juice mixed with Witchhazel can also be used as a conditioning massage. As a final rinse after washing hair, a tablespoonful of Cider Vinegar will restore the pH balance.

Aromatherapy Oils

★ *Scalp tonic:*   add one drop of Rosemary, one drop of Thyme and one drop of Sage to an eggcupful of Almond or Soya oil. Massage into hair prior to washing and leave on for a good ten minutes.

DIARRHOEA

A bout of diarrhoea can range from mildly uncomfortable to totally uncontrollable. It all depends on the viciousness of the bug that causes the infection. The bugs responsible for diarrhoea attach themselves to the intestine and prompt quick evacuation of faeces when they are still in a watery state. The main causes of infection are viruses, such as gastroenteritis, and bacteria, such as listeria food poisoning, irritation from drugs, parasites, food allergy, stress and bad diet.

Diet

★ *AVOID*   overloading the digestive system when suffering from diarrhoea.

★ *EAT*   nutritional but plain foods such as lightly steamed vegetables and brown rice, as well as home made vegetable soups. Live yogurt helps put back beneficial bacteria into the intestine which has been lost by the stomach upset – some yogurts actually contain extra portions of good lactobacillus acidophilus bacteria, so look out for those. Diarrhoea dehydrates the body very quickly, so DRINK PLENTY of liquid.

| Beneficial Supplements |

Lactobacillus acidophilus supplements, from health food stores
Vitamin B Complex (up to 100 mg daily)

| Homoeopathy |

Chosen remedy to be taken every half hour over a five-hour period.
Arsenicum 6c: for severe diarrhoea, with mucus, as well as vomiting
Rhus Tox 6c: with blood and mucus
Podophyllum 6c: mucus, green colour, worse in morning
Veratrum 6c: vomiting, as well as cold sweat

| Herbal Remedies |

★ *Infusion:*　　(for tea) Slippery Elm, Golden Seal and Meadowsweet. Combine two parts of Slippery Elm to one part each of Golden Seal and Meadowsweet, add one teaspoon of the mixture to a teapot, cover with a cupful of boiling water, infuse for ten minutes then drink.

★ *Herbal drink:*　Slippery Elm in particular is a time-honoured remedy for all forms of stomach upset, take one teaspoon of Slippery Elm powder in a glass of hot water, three times daily.

| Aromatherapy Oils |

★ *Massage oil:*　add one drop each of Savory, Lavender, Ginger and Orange Blossom to an eggcupful of Almond or Soya oil, massage into the abdomen.

DIZZINESS AND FAINTING

Dizziness is associated with an imbalance in the body's balancing mechanism. It can be caused by stress, low blood sugar, low blood pressure, vertigo or a stomach upset. Symptoms that often occur with it are nausea, heavy perspiration and pallor.

Fainting occurs when the blood supply to the brain is lowered and gathers elsewhere, often in the stomach or legs. As soon as the head is brought level with the heart, the patient will revive. Fainting can be the result of shock or standing up quickly from a sedentary position.

Diet

★ *AVOID*　　　　refined sugar products which give you an instant energy boost, but then leave your blood sugar low again.

★ *EAT*　　　　little and often, particularly foods rich in Vitamins B6 and B3. These include brewer's yeast, organ meats, green leafy vegetables (cabbage in particular), milk, wholegrains, nuts, fish, eggs, dates and figs.

Beneficial Supplements

Vitamin B6 (50–100 g daily)
Vitamin B3 (also known as Niacin, 50–100 g daily)
Manganese (in a multi-vitamin and mineral tablet)
Bach Flower Rescue Remedy (a couple of drops to help to revive, from health food stores)

Homoeopathy

Chosen remedy to be taken when symptoms appear – up to ten doses per day.
China 6c: nausea, blood loss, dizziness

Pulsatilla 6c: dizziness in hot, stuffy room
Arnica 6c: dizziness from sudden movements
Aconite 6c: fainting from fear or emotional excitement
Arsenicum 6c: fainting while agitated, cold

Herbal Remedies

★ *Infusion:*   (for tea) Peppermint. Add one heaped teaspoon of Peppermint to a teapot, cover with a cupful of boiling water, leave to infuse for five minutes then drink.

★ *Reviver:*   place a little St John's Wort oil on a ball of cotton wool, hold under nose to stimulate senses.

Aromatherapy Oils

★ *Massage oil:*   Caraway, add three drops to an egg-cupful of Almond or Soya oil, massage into temples, cheeks and neck.

EARACHE

Earache is a common problem among children and can be linked to a sore throat and toothache. When the eardrum becomes inflamed, it is very painful, can produce pus, and is usually due to infection. With an infected ear, it also becomes more difficult to hear, to speak without ears popping, and to balance.

It is important to keep the affected ear out of draughts and the patient generally warm. Any persistent and painful earache should be shown to your GP as, although rare, it can be quite serious.

Diet

★ *AVOID*   dairy products which are mucus-forming if the earache is linked to flu or a cold.

★ *DRINK PLENTY* of liquids, as earache is often associated with a blockage in the Eustachian tube (which runs from the nose to the ear), and a throat infection.

★ *EAT*   foods rich in Vitamin C such as rosehip syrup, blackcurrants, kale, broccoli, citrus fruits and cabbage to help fight any infection.

Beneficial Supplements

Vitamin C (1 g daily)
Vitamin A (5000 IU daily)
Vitamin B Complex (up to 100 g daily)
Zinc (15 mg daily)

Homoeopathy

Chosen remedy to be taken three times a day over one week.
Hepar Sulph 6c: ear throbs, warmth soothes
Pulsatilla 6c: possible discharge, patient upset and desires company
Belladonna 6c: sore throat, headache, throbbing ache in ears

Herbal Remedies

★ *Infusion:*   (for tea) Chamomile, Lobelia and Echinacea. Combine equal parts of the herbs, then add one heaped teaspoon to a teapot, cover with a cupful of boiling water, infuse for ten minutes then drink. Twice daily.

| Aromatherapy Oils |

★ *Undiluted application:* gently tip one to two drops of Mullein, Garlic or Cajuput into the affected ears three times a day to help to soothe and disinfect the inflammation. Alternatively, the oils can be added to a piece of cotton wool, which is then stuck gently into the outer ear.

ECZEMA

Eczema is often used as a blanket term for varying skin conditions. Severity can differ from person to person but generally, eczema results in red, itchy skin – sometimes puffy, scaliness and blisters. It can affect babies, children and adults. It often erupts around the hands, wrists and elbows. The neck and face are also common sites of irritation.

Eczema is not contagious but seems to have a hereditary link, those prone to asthma, hayfever and other allergies may well develop it. Eczema can be irritated by such substances as detergents, rubber, metal and paints. Stress and emotional upsets can also act as eczema triggers.

| Diet |

★ *AVOID* dairy products, particularly cow's milk and processed foods with chemical additives (it can provoke an allergic reaction).

★ *INSTEAD DRINK* soya milk products and plenty of fresh foods, avoiding chocolate, coffee and tea.

★ *EAT* wheatgerm which contains Vitamin E, Gamma Linolenic Acid (GLA), which some eczema sufferers are deficient in, and Vitamins B1, B2, B3, B5 and B6, all good for skin. Wheatgerm can easily be added to cereals.

Beneficial Supplements

Oil of Evening Primrose (2 x 500 mg daily)
Vitamin B Complex (up to 100 mg daily)
or
Brewer's yeast (six tablets daily)

Homoeopathy

Chosen remedy to be taken three times daily over two weeks.
Sulphur 6c: itching, red skin, aggravated by water
Graphites 6c: eczema on scalp
Rhus Tox 6c: dry eczema on hands and wrists, scabs
Petroleum 6c: eczema causes skin to crack

Herbal Remedies

★ ***Decoction:*** (for tea) Burdock root, Yellow Dock root and Sarsaparilla. Combine equal parts and put 25 g (1 oz) of mixture into a saucepan (not aluminium) containing 900 ml (1½ pints) boiling water. Simmer for ten minutes, strain and drink a cup at a time, three times daily.

★ ***Skin application:*** apply Calendula (Marigold) lotion. Bathe sore patches with an infusion of Witchhazel 25 g (1 oz) herb to 600 ml (1 pint) boiling water and infuse for ten minutes.

Aromatherapy Oils

★ ***Massage oil:*** add one drop each of Juniper,

Geranium and Lavender to an egg-cupful of Almond or Soya oil. Massage into affected area. Alternatively, use Chamomile, Hyssop and Sage together.

FLATULENCE

Wind in the stomach and intestines is an uncomfortable and embarrassing problem. A build-up of excess gas and air in the stomach can be caused by several things: some foods such as pulses and rich food, eating too fast, drinking while eating, talking while eating, and fermentation in the stomach due to an over-complement of bad bacteria living in the gut. Bad posture and lack of exercise can also contribute to the problem. In some cases, the stomach becomes bloated and twinges of pain can be felt.

Diet

★ *AVOID* wolfing down food, make sure it is chewed properly before entering your stomach so that it is easy to digest. If you suffer frequently from wind, food in your stomach may be fermenting, in which case do not worsen the situation by mixing carbohydrates with proteins – eat them separately. An imbalance of bad bacteria in the stomach can be supplemented by good bacteria through eating live yogurt. Wind in the stomach can be absorbed by eating vegetable charcoal biscuits (black in colour!). Garlic is an excellent tool in digestion and should be eaten raw or cooked in your meals.

Beneficial Supplements

Brewer's yeast (six tablets daily)
Hydrochloric Acid tablets: your doctor may advise you to supplement your diet with these if you suffer from fermentation in the stomach, caused by too little pepsin and gastric hydrochloric acid.

Homoeopathy

Chosen remedy to be taken every half hour up to ten doses per day.
Carbo Veg 6c: wind in upper abdomen
Nux Vomica 6c: for flatulence associated with constipation
Lycopodium 6c: wind in lower abdomen

Herbal Remedies

★ *Infusion:*   (for tea) Aniseed, Fennel and Coriander. Combine equal parts and steep 25 g (1 oz) in 600 ml (1 pint) of boiling water for ten minutes, then drink two to three cups daily. A tea can also be prepared using Peppermint, drink after meals. Cardamom seeds can be chewed as a preventive measure.

Aromatherapy Oils

★ *Massage oil:*   add one drop each of Aniseed, Caraway, Ginger and Rosemary to an eggcupful of Almond or Soya oil. Massage into the abdomen.

FLU

Flu is a virus infection, and there are many different types of virus floating around. However, once you have had one strain you will never suffer from it again as the immune system produces antibodies against it.

Although the virus essentially attacks the respiratory tract, the symptoms of flu are much more widespread. Flu can manifest itself in aching limbs, fever, cough, inflammation of the mucous membranes, diarrhoea, vomiting, fatigue and slight depression. It is a very contagious disease and takes up to four days to incubate, so as soon as you feel the symptoms coming on, go straight to bed, keep warm and don't give it to all your colleagues.

Diet

At the onset of flu, the appetite is suppressed and the patient NEEDS a large intake of fluids. To give the body strength to fight the virus, the fluids should be as nutritious as possible. A homemade vegetable or meat broth is ideal and should be consumed alongside PLENTY of fruit juices (particulary citrus for their Vitamin C value), herb teas, and lemon, honey and hot water. If possible, use freshly squeezed fruit juices which retain far more of their goodness than processed juices. When the appetite returns to normal, EAT plain food, full of protein which is needed by the body's recovery mechanism. Combine fish, white meat, soya protein or tofu with lightly cooked vegetables, baked potatoes and brown rice.

Beneficial Supplements

Vitamin C (2 g daily)
Spirulina algae (packed with protein)
Vitamin B Complex (up to 100 g daily)
Vitamin A (5000 IU)

Homoeopathy

Chosen remedy to be taken every two hours up to ten doses per day.

Arsenicum 6c: fatigue, can't move around, fever, diarrhoea

Bryonia 30c: dry mouth, cough, can't move around

Nux Vomica 6c: at onset of flu – aches and pains, fatigue

Phytolacca 6c: swollen glands, pain in ears

Herbal Remedies

★ **Infusion:** (for tea) Boneset, Peppermint and Elderflower. Combine equal parts, add one heaped teaspoon to a teapot, cover with a cupful of boiling water, infuse for ten minutes and drink, twice daily. It will promote sweating and help to rid the body of the virus. Yarrow tea is useful at the beginning of flu (one teaspoon dried herb to one cup of water). Add a little honey and Cayenne to it.

Aromatherapy Oils

★ **Inhalant:** add three drops of Eucalyptus and three drops of Pine to a bowl of steaming hot water and inhale the vapours.

★ **Massage oil:** Combine one drop each of Lemon, Sage, Thyme and Hyssop to an egg-cupful of Almond or Soya oil, massage into the chest.

GINGIVITIS

According to the British Dental Association, gingivitis causes the loss of more teeth than tooth decay.

Gingivitis is an inflammation of the gums, caused by bacteria. The gums become swollen, soft and may bleed.

The mouth is full of bacteria, normally harmless, but sometimes the bacteria manage to infiltrate the gums through the scaly build-up around teeth called tartar. Tartar is a mixture between plaque (deposits of food) and calcium from the saliva. If the tartar is allowed to build up around the teeth, gingivitis can develop. The gums recede and the bony socket around the tooth is destroyed, so that eventually the tooth will have to be removed to stop the infection.

This is the reason it is so important to see a dentist regularly and to brush teeth after every meal or snack. Use dental floss around teeth to stop the collection of tartar.

Diet

★ **EAT PLENTY** — of crunchy food such as raw carrots, apples, pears, raw white cabbage, lightly cooked broccoli and cabbage, which all act as an abrasive and do not harm the teeth.

★ *AVOID* — refined sugar products, because they actually ferment in the mouth, turning into acids that attack the teeth, promoting plaque and bacterial growth. Chocolates, toffees, biscuits, iced buns, canned drinks and sweets should be avoided.

Beneficial Supplements

Vitamin A (500–1200 IU)
Vitamin B6 (50 mg daily)
Rosehip Syrup (Vitamin C)

| Homoeopathy |

Chosen remedy to be taken three times daily up to ten doses per day.

Hepar Sulph 6c: to calm the infection

Mercurius 6c: severe gingivitis, bad breath

Natrum Mur 6c: sensitive teeth, prone to ulcers, swollen gums

| Herbal Remedies |

★ *Mouthwash:*   Echineacea, Eucalyptus and Myrrh. Combine equal parts of the herbs and add 25 g (1 oz) to 600 ml (1 pint) boiling water, infuse for ten minutes, then strain. Rinse with the mouthwash every time you clean your teeth.

| Aromatherapy Oils |

★ *Mouthwash:*   add one drop of Sage, one drop of Myrrh and one drop of Fennel to a glass of warm water and gargle. Alternatively, rub a little Myrrh diluted in warm water on the affected gums.

HAYFEVER

Every year, an estimated two million people in Britain sniff and sneeze their way through the summer months. The cause is hayfever, an allergic response to flower, tree and grass pollens. When these minute particles of pollen are breathed in, the body's immune system wrongly assumes that these particles are harmful and produces histamine to fight them off. Histamine triggers the manufacture of excessive mucus, which can turn into catarrh, and causes watery eyes, sneezing, coughing, itchy skin and headaches. The hayfever sufferer often has a family history of asthma and other allergies.

However, hayfever is not necessarily a lifelong allergy: some people suddenly develop it in their adulthood. This could be due to a build-up of unnecessary chemicals in the body, which trigger a pollen allergy.

Diet

★ *AVOID*   mucus forming foods such as dairy products, chocolate, tea and coffee. Avoid processed food with additional chemical additives, as these can add to the toxic build-up in your body and contribute towards forming catarrh.

★ *EAT PLENTY*   of unrefined starchy foods such as potatoes, brown rice, wholemeal bread, and wholewheat pasta rather than buns, cakes and fried foods.

Beneficial Supplements

Vitamin B Complex (up to 100 mg daily)
Vitamin C (2 g daily)
or
Rosehip Syrup (Vitamin C).

Homoeopathy

Chosen remedy to be taken over two days up to ten doses per day.
Allium Cepa 6c: itchy nose and eyes, watery mucus
Mixed Pollen 6c: for all types of hayfever
Sabadilla 6c: headache and sneezing, watery mucus
Kali Carb 6c: chronic catarrh, depression
Nux Vomica 6c: sensitive eyes, itching between throat and ears

Herbal Remedies

★ *Infusion:*   (for tea) Elderflower and Golden Rod. Combine equal parts of the two herbs, then add 25 g (1 oz) of mixture to 600 ml (1 pint) boiling water. Infuse for ten minutes, strain and drink three times daily. An infusion of Lavender and Thyme could also help.

★ *Infusion:* (for eye bath) Witchhazel and Eyebright. Make an infusion and soak compress of linen or gauze in warm liquid, apply to closed eyes for five minutes.

Aromatherapy Oils

★ *Inhalant:* add two drops of Hyssop and three drops of Pine to a bowl of steaming water. Cover head with towel and breathe in steam for five minutes.

HEADACHES AND MIGRAINES

These can range from a minor irritation to a searing pain. Migraine is a particularly bad form of headache, which some people seem more susceptible to than others. Most ordinary headaches are caused by muscle tension, tiredness and anxiety, but the headache can also be a sign of another health problem such as, 'flu, low blood sugar, diabetes or hypertension. These kind of headaches can be helped away with massage, and the Alexander Technique, if the reason for your continued headaches is bad posture.

In the case of migraine, the headache has something to do with the expansion of the blood vessels in the tissue surrounding the brain, but experts are still uncertain as to the real causes. Those suffering from a migraine attack can't stand bright light and often feel nauseous. The attack comes on suddenly and violently, often forcing the sufferer to retire to bed.

Diet

Natural substances in some foods actually trigger a migraine attack (tyramine, phenylethamine and octopamine). Foods containing these substances include chocolate, caffeine, cheese and dairy products, fatty and fried foods, pork, onions, citrus fruits and alcohol. Try not eating them and see what happens. The key is to eat little and often to keep blood sugar constant, and the best way to do this is on a wholefood diet.

Beneficial Supplements

Vitamin B Complex (30 mg daily)
Vitamin B3 (50 mg daily)
Vitamin B6 (50 mg daily)
Calcium (100 mg daily)
Ginseng (for stress headache)

Homoeopathy

Headaches:
Chosen remedy to be taken as often as necessary up to ten doses per day.
Aconite 30c: congested feeling, throbbing
Nux Vomica 6c: splitting headache, dizziness
Pulsatilla 6c: throbbing, goes in waves, indigestion
Arnica 6c: ache at the front of the head, made worse by movement

Migraines:
Chosen remedy to be taken as often as needed up to ten doses per day.
Pulsatilla 6c: bursting feeling in head
Spigelia 6c: left-sided headache, palpitations
Natrum Mur 6c: throbbing on top of head
Sanguinaria 6c: right-sided, pain begins at back of head

Herbal Remedies

★ **Infusion:** (for tea) Lavender, Rosemary and Marjoram. Combine equal parts of the herbs, take one teaspoon and add to a cup of boiling water. Infuse for ten minutes, strain and then drink.

★ **Bath soak:** to a warm bath add some fresh Lavender, let the aroma soothe an aching head

★ **Migraine:** Feverfew tablets are very beneficial, available from health food stores.

Aromatherapy Oils

★ **Massage oil:** (for headache) mix one drop each of Lemon, Eucalyptus, Aniseed and Lavender to an eggcupful of Almond oil and massage into temples.

★ **Massage oil:** (for migraine) mix one drop each of Basil, Aniseed (good for nauseous feelings) and Melissa to an eggcupful of Almond oil and massage into temples.

INDIGESTION

Indigestion is one of the commonest complaints around and one which it is easy to do something about. Indigestion can produce flatulence, stomach pains, nausea and headaches. It can be caused by a gastric ulcer or gastritis but this is rare: the usual problem is over-eating, eating too fast, eating the wrong kinds of food, heavy smoking, fermentation of food in the stomach (see page 28) or anxiety.

Diet

First of all, slow down your rate of eating. Improved posture may also help.

★ *DO NOT*   mix starchy foods with proteins, or fruits and vegetables – eat them separately.

★ *AVOID*   fried and fatty foods, which are difficult to digest.

★ *EAT PLENTY*   of garlic as this helps with the digestive process. Older people with frequent indigestion could be suffering from lack of digestive enzymes: a simple way to reverse this is to eat fresh pineapple which is full of these enzymes. Vegetable charcoal biscuits help absorb excess gas in the stomach.

Beneficial Supplements

Garlic capsules (at least two daily)
Brewer's yeast (six tablets daily)
Bromelain or papain (pineapple and papaya) tablets

Homoeopathy

Chosen remedy to be taken every half hour for up to ten doses per day.
Nux Vomica 6c: heartburn, flatulence, constipation, excessive eating
Carbo Veg 6c: indigestion in upper abdomen, nausea, flatulence
Sulphur 6c: chronic indigestion
Natrum Mur 6c: stress and anxiety–related

Herbal Remedies

★ *Infusion:*   (for tea) Peppermint or Chamomile. Add one heaped teaspoon of either herb to a cupful of boiling water, infuse for ten minutes, strain and then drink. Bay Leaves, Basil, Ginger, Sage or Thyme added to food aid digestion.

Aromatherapy Oils

★ *Massage oil:*   combine one drop each of Basil, Melissa, Thyme and Clove to one eggcupful of Almond or Soya oil and rub into the abdomen. Alternatively, add two drops each to a warm bath.

INFLUENZA *see* FLU

INSECT BITES

Bee, wasp and insect bites are enough to ruin any holiday, particularly if it's very hot and the stings swell up or itch unmercifully.

Diet

There's not a lot you can eat to ward off insect bites. However, you can apply vinegar or lemon juice (acid) to a wasp sting and bicarbonate of soda (alkaline) to a bee sting to reduce the pain and swelling.

Beneficial Supplements

Vitamin B1 (75–100 mg daily one week before and during holiday)

Homoeopathy

Chosen remedy to be taken every quarter hour for up to ten doses per day.
Apis 6c: for bee or mosquito stings

Ledum 6c: painful sting but not so red and swollen
Hypercal mother tincture: apply to the sting to reduce inflammation.

Homoeopathically prepared iodine tablets can act as an insect repellent.

| Herbal Remedies |

★ *Skin application:* rub affected area with Calendula (Marigold) cream for an antiseptic, soothing effect.

| Aromatherapy Oils |

★ *Massage oil:* (repellent) add fifteen drops each of Basil and Peppermint to 50 ml (2 fl oz) of Almond oil, rub over exposed areas of the body.

★ *Skin application:* (post sting) add two drops each of Lavender, Cajuput and Tea Tree to an eggcupful of Almond or Soya oil, rub on to sting and surrounding area.

INSOMNIA

Insomnia is a troublesome problem to suffer from and can be a result of pain, indigestion or sheer anxiety and nervous tension. Although scientists don't know exactly why, everybody needs the amount of sleep right for them, the average is about eight hours. Without sufficient sleep we become irritable and sluggish, and sometimes ill.

| Diet |

★ *AVOID* drinking coffee or tea during the couple of hours before bedtime as caffeine is a stimulant. Do not eat a heavy meal just before bedtime, as the digestive system will have to start up again.

★ **EAT**   foods rich in the amino-acid tryptophan, these include starchy foods such as bread, pasta, rice, cakes, breakfast cereals and potatoes.

Beneficial Supplements

Calcium (up to 1000 mg daily)
Magnesium (up to 200 mg daily).

Homoeopathy

Chosen remedy to be taken three times daily over two weeks.

Lycopodium 6c: anxious, unable to get off to sleep, then feel very sleepy in the morning
Coffea 6c: over-excitement, too much coffee
Cocculus 6c: over-tired, mind still active
Passiflora 6c: restless sleep
Chamomilla 6c: excellent remedy for children

Herbal Remedies

★ *Infusion:*   (for tea) Balm, Passiflora and Wild Lettuce. Combine equal parts of all three herbs, add one teaspoon to a cupful of boiling water, infuse for ten minutes, strain then drink just before bedtime. If you are suffering from a lot of nervous tension, add some Scullcap to the recipe. A herbal pillow could also help send you off to sleep.

Aromatherapy Oils

★ *Massage oil:*   add two drops of Basil, one drop of Chamomile, one drop of Sandalwood and one drop of Ylang Ylang to an eggcupful of Almond or Soya oil. Massage into the body before going to bed.

★ *Bath soak:* add two drops of each of the above oils to warm the bath.

MOUTH ULCERS

Mouth ulcers are sore, irritating blisters that occur on the tongue, the gums or the inside of the cheeks. They can be an indication of ill health, stress or a tooth that is rubbing either on the tongue or the cheeks. Sometimes they erupt singly, at other times they come in crops which can be very painful for the sufferer.

| Diet |

If your ulcers are due to anxiety, stress or bad diet, you can greatly help by making sure you EAT PLENTY of foods containing Vitamin A and B2 which help keep the mucous membranes healthy. Vitamin A foods include liver, butter, eggs, fish and fish oils, cheese, carrots, dark green vegetables such as spinach, broccoli and cabbage, plus peaches and apricots. Vitamin B2 foods include wholegrains, wheatgerm, sprouting seeds, fish, red meat and green leafy vegetables.

| Beneficial Supplements |

Vitamin A (4000 IU daily)
Vitamin B2 (10 mg daily)

| Homoeopathy |

Chosen remedy to be taken four times daily over five days.
Mercurius 6c: tongue ulcers, stinging
Calendula tincture: applied sparingly to the ulcer.

| Herbal Remedies |

★ *Infusion:*   (for mouthwash) Myrrh, Red Sage or Chamomile. Add one heaped teaspoon of chosen herb to a cupful of boiling water, infuse for ten minutes, then swill round the mouth and spit out. Do this three times daily.

| Aromatherapy Oils |

★ *Mouthwash:*   add two drops of either Lemon, Tea Tree or Myrrh to an eggcupful of warm water. Swill around mouth and spit out.

MENSTRUAL PROBLEMS

AMENORRHOEA (DELAYED OR ABSENT PERIODS)

Primary amenorrhoea applies to girls who have not yet started their periods or women who have just gone through the menopause. Secondary amenorrhoea is when women of childbearing age stop having periods. Apart from becoming pregnant, periods can also cease when a woman comes off the Pill, does a lot of physical exercise, or is under considerable stress.

| Diet |

★ *EAT*   a basic wholefood diet with plenty of fruit and vegetables, raw and lightly cooked, wholegrains, fish, white meat, wholemeal bread, some eggs and cheese, pulses and sprouting seeds. In this way the body receives an all-round diet full of essential nutrients which the body may be lacking to function correctly.

Beneficial Supplements

Vitamin B Complex (up to 100 mg daily)
Zinc (up to 15 mg daily)
Magnesium (up to 200 mg)
Vitamin C (500 mg daily)
Vitamin E (50–200 IU daily)
Manganese (3–5 mg daily)

Homoeopathy

Chosen remedy to be taken twice daily over two weeks.
Pulsatilla 30c: usually irregular
Ignatia 30c: emotional upset
Calcarea 30c: anaemic, nerves on edge
Natrum Mur 30c: irritable, constipation, emotional upset

Herbal Remedies

★ **Infusion:**   (for tea) Pennyroyal, Tansy and Southernwood. Combine equal parts of the herbs then add one teaspoon of the mixture to a cupful of boiling water, infuse for ten minutes, strain and drink. Drink twice daily for one week.

Aromatherapy Oils

★ **Massage oil:**   add three drops each of Tarragon, Sage, Chamomile and Thyme to 50 ml (2 fl oz) of Almond or Soya oil. Rub into the abdomen and lower back.

★ **Bath soak:**   add two drops each of above oils to a warm bath.

DYSMENORRHOEA (PAINFUL PERIODS)

Painful periods are a very common state of affairs in teenage girls and young women. Usually the problem clears with age, or after birth of a child, but it can persist for quite a few years before the pains subside. Pains include lower back ache, stomach cramps, a sense of fragility around the stomach, and sometimes vomiting.

This uncomfortable reaction to the onset of a period is thought to be caused by an imbalance of sex hormones or an over-emotional state. A hot water bottle against the back or stomach can help to relieve symptoms.

Diet

As in Amenorrhoea, a good basic wholefood diet is vital. Sprinkle wheatgerm on to your breakfast cereal, as it is high in the beneficial gamma linolenic acid. Safflower, Soya and Sunflower oils are rich sources of linoleic acid – again important in the functioning of the reproductive organs. Try to cook with these instead of animal fat or plain 'vegetable' oil.

Beneficial Supplements

Oil of Evening Primrose (2 x 500 mg daily a week before and during your period).

Homoeopathy

Chosen remedy to be taken every half hour for up to ten doses per day.

Pulsatilla 30c: localized pains, vomiting, backache
Gelsemium 30c: aches and shooting pains in the abdomen and lower back
Chamomilla 30c: stomach cramps
Viburnum 30c: pain in thighs

Herbal Remedies

★ *Infusion:*   (for tea) Cramp Bark. Add one tea-spoon to a cupful of boiling water, infuse for 10 minutes, strain then drink. Take three times a day during period.

Aromatherapy Oils

★ *Massage oil:*   choose a combination of three oils from Rosemary, Sage, Tarragon, Thyme, Jasmine and Cypress. Add two drops of each to an eggcupful of Almond or Soya oil, rub into the abdomen, thighs and back.

PRE-MENSTRUAL SYNDROME (PMS)

PMS is suffered by 40 per cent of women. It usually strikes during the ten days before a period and can involve physical symptoms such as tender breasts, water retention, fatigue, spots, diarrhoea and constipation.

The mental syptoms can be more disturbing such as depression, severe irritability and emotional behaviour. The cause is thought to be a hormone imbalance.

Diet

★ *AVOID*   alcohol, refined sugar products and fatty foods which use up the body's supply of B Vitamins – these vitamins aid the correct functioning of menstruation.

★ *EAT*   a wholefood diet with foods essentially rich in Vitamin B6, such as wheatgerm, liver, oats, nuts, brown rice and bananas.

Beneficial Supplements

Brewer's yeast (six tablets daily)
Vitamin B6 (up to 50 mg daily)
Oil of Evening Primrose (2 x 500 mg capsules daily)

Homoeopathy

Chosen remedy to be taken twice daily during three days before the onset of PMS.

Lycopodium 30c: ill–tempered, depression, craving sweet foods

Natrum Mur 30c: fluid retention, melancholic, irritable

Pulsatilla 30c: stomach upset, tearful

Calcarea 30c: over-tired and clumsy

Herbal Remedies

Agnus Castus (one teaspoon to a mug of water) three times daily, a week to ten days before your period.

Aromatherapy Oils

★ *Massage oil:*   add three drops of Parsley, two drops of Neroli and two drops of Clary-Sage to an eggcupful of Almond or Soya oil and massage into the abdomen.

★ *Bath soak:*   add three drops of each oil to a warm bath.

PILES (Haemorrhoids)

Piles can be internal and external. They are distended veins in or around the rectum. The internal condition is termed a haemorrhoid, the classic symptom of which is bleeding. Long term sufferers of haemorrhoids are often anaemic.

Haemorrhoids should always be investigated by a doctor as they can be a sign of cancer of the rectum. Doctors tend to refer to Piles as the small blood blisters situated around the anus, which are relatively easy to banish.

Diet

Both haemorroids and piles can be caused by constipation and overstraining as a result.

★ *AVOID*   highly refined foods that lack fibre, cut down on meat that takes a long time to digest and can sit around in the bowel.

★ *EAT*   a diet full of fibre and roughage, that will slip through the bowels with ease. Fibrous foods include wheat bran, wholemeal flour, brown rice, green-leaved vegetables, dried fruit and pulses.

Beneficial Supplements

Vitamin C (500 mg daily)
Rutin (100 mg daily)
Vitamin B Complex (up to 100 mg daily)
Vitamin B6 (10 mg daily if bleeding occurs)

Homoeopathy

Chosen remedy to be taken four times a day over a week.
Sulphur 6c: itching, redness, constipation
Collinsonia 6c: bleeding, itching, constipation
Aesculus 6c: passing stools brings about splintery sensation, hot burning feeling
Aloe 6c: burning sensation, piles like small bunch of grapes, diarrhoea

Herbal Remedies

★ *Infusion:*   (for tea) Lady's Mantle. Add one teaspoon to one cupful of boiling water, infuse for ten minutes, strain and drink twice daily.

★ *Ointment:*   a handful of bruised Periwinkle leaves added to 25 g (1 oz) of melted vaseline and left to cool can be applied. The same can be done with Witchhazel.

Aromatherapy Oils

★ *Bath soak:*   add three drops each of Cypress, Myrrh and Juniper oils to a warm bath.

SORE THROAT AND TONSILLITIS

The throat is often the first part of the body to be affected if the immune system is at a low ebb. A sore throat can be the body's way of saying it has had enough and needs a rest. Inflammation of the throat can also be a result of a viral infection such as tonsillitis, laryngitis or a cold and can be accompanied by headaches, a temperature and fatigue.

In the specific case of tonsillitis, the tonsils become inflamed when attacked by bacteria. In a healthy body they act as a channel through which flows lymph, a substance that assists in expelling toxins. If the body is suffering from an overload of these toxins, the strain may well manifest itself in the tonsils.

Diet

★ *AVOID*   any processed foods, coffee, tea and chocolate and mucus forming dairy foods except yogurt.

★ *DRINK PLENTY*   of liquids, particularly citrus fruit juices which help to tighten mucous membranes, making it easier to breathe.

★ *EAT PLENTY*   of protein to bolster your immune system (pulses, a little lean meat, soya foods, hard cheese, milk).

★ *EAT*   foods containing Vitamin B5 (liver, eggs, green leafy vegetables, nuts and wheatgerm).

Beneficial Supplements

Vitamin B5 (50 mg daily)
Folic Acid (200 mcg)
Vitamin B6 (up to 50 mg daily)
Vitamin C (2 g daily during infection)

Homoeopathy

Chosen remedy to be taken every two hours up to ten doses per day.
Belladonna 6c: feverish, sore throat
Aconite 30c: swollen tonsils, congestion, dryness, burning sensation
Hepar Sulph 6c: irritable, chilliness, enlarged glands, feels as though something is stuck in throat
Gelsemium 6c: difficulty in swallowing, pain in neck and ears

Herbal Remedies

★ *Infusion:*   (for tea or gargle) Red Sage. Add one teaspoon of the herb to a cupful of boiling water, infuse for ten minutes, strain and then drink or gargle. Do this three times daily.

Aromatherapy Oils

★ *Inhalation:*   add five drops of Eucalyptus to a bowl of hot water, cover head with towel and inhale.

★ *Gargle:*   add three drops of either Lemon or
Tea Tree to a glass of warm water,
gargle and spit out after use.

STRESS

Stress is a much talked about phenomenon these days
and can manifest itself in different ways. Many doctors
now believe that stress can be an indirect cause of
illness.

When you find yourself in a stressful situation, the
body immediately goes into the fight or flight response,
adrenalin starts to pump and you are prepared for
action. If there is no outlet for these feelings, you can
literally start to burn out, leading to frayed nerves,
irritability, depression and fatigue.

Minor and major health problems – such as heart
attacks, stomach ulcers, aches and pains, diarrhoea, sore
throat and dry or spotty skin can all be linked to stress.
However, even if you do have a hectic, difficult life, a
build up of stress can be released.

Endeavour to have at least three forty-minute periods
of hard exercise every week, such as cycling, aerobics,
dance, squash or football. Relaxation techniques are
very valuable, and once learnt, they can be used
anywhere, anytime. Learn these techniques at your local
evening class or buy an appropriate tape or a book from
your local health food store. Many people also find
meditation helpful.

Diet

Foods rich in Vitamin C and Vitamin B Complex will
help keep the effects of stress at bay.

★ *EAT PLENTY*   of citrus fruits, lightly steamed green
leafy vegetables, blackcurrants, sprout-

ing seeds, wholegrains, wheatgerm, liver, kidney and heart. Oats have a very calming effect on the nerves so eat a bowl of porridge daily.

★ *AVOID*   eating refined carbohydrate foods (white flour and white sugar products) as they use up the de-stressing B Vitamins during digestion.

Beneficial Supplements

Vitamin B Complex (up to 100 mg daily)
Vitamin C (1 g daily)
Vitamin B6 (25 mg daily for mild depression)

Homoeopathy

Chosen remedy to be taken every six hours over two weeks.
Ignatia 30c: stress following emotional upset
Piric Ac 30c: due to overwork
Phosphoric Ac: due to grief or bad news

Herbal Remedies

★ *Infusion:*   (for tea) Damiana and Scullcap. Combine equal parts of the herbs and add one teaspoon to a cup of boiling water, infuse for ten minutes, strain then drink. Drink once a day over short periods of stress, towards the end of day.

Aromatherapy Oils

★ *Massage oil:*   add two drops of Basil, and one drop each of Neroli, Cedarwood and Juniper to an eggcupful of Almond or Soya oil. Massage into the body before retiring for the night.

SUNBURN

Sunburn is caused by over-exposure to the sun's rays, often not visible until an hour or two after exposure. The cells which produce the pigment melanin are unable to cope with the amount of sun pouring on to the skin, so instead of going brown, the skin burns and turns a pinky/red colour. The skin becomes dehydrated and will eventually peel off. Severe sunburn can be the cause of sunstroke – a very unpleasant illness with severe headache, diarrhoea, sickness and fever.

Continued over-exposure to the sun ages the skin. To avoid permanent damage, cover yourself with a generous layer of suntan lotion (at least Factor Eight) when sunbathing.

Diet

★ *EAT PLENTY*   of foods containing Vitamin C to help heal skin once it has been burnt, such as blackcurrants, broccoli, kale, sprouts, citrus fruits, sprouting seeds and watercress.

Beneficial Supplements

Vitamin A (600 IU daily)
Vitamin C (1 g daily)
Vitamin E (100 IU daily)
Vitamin E cream: apply directly to the burnt skin

Homoeopathy

Chosen remedy to be taken every half hour for up to ten doses per day.
Belladonna 6c: for a touch of sunstroke
Glonoin 30c: severe sunstroke
Sol 30c: to prevent sunburn – every four hours while in strong sunlight.

Herbal Remedies

★ *Skin applications:* apply Aloe Vera gel straight to the skin to cool and soothe. Calendula lotion is also helpful.

Aromatherapy Oils

★ *Skin application:* Lavender oil applied directly to the burnt area – but use sparingly.

THRUSH (vaginal)

Thrush is an infection of any of the mucous membranes, but particularly the vagina and mouth, with the yeast fungus called *candida albicans*. In a healthy body, candida is controlled by beneficial bacteria.

When these good bacteria are reduced by bad nutrition or antibiotics, they can no longer contain the candida yeast. It runs riot and manifests itself as white patches on the tongue or vagina. Vaginal thrush causes itching and discomfort.

Diet

★ *AVOID* eating too many acid-forming foods such as meat, fish, nuts, bread, yeast, grains, butter, cheese, eggs and chocolate. Instead eat more aikaline-forming foods such as fruit and vegetables, soya products, milk and yogurt.

★ *EAT PLENTY* of live natural yogurt which contains good bacteria (lactobacillus acidophilus) which re-colonize the gut and help to re-establish control over candida. Live yogurt can also be inserted into the vagina, using a tampon.

| Beneficial Supplements |

Garlic perles
Vitamin B Complex (up to 100 mg daily)

| Homoeopathy |

Chosen remedy to be taken six times daily for up to five days.
Pulsatilla 6c: opaque discharge, sore, worse before and after periods
Aconitum Napellus 6c: dry, hot and sensitive vagina
Sulphur 6c: creamy discharge, stings, aching in abdomen
Alumina 6c: yellow discharge, itchyness, worse before and after periods

| Herbal Remedies |

★ *Infusion:* (for swabbing) Golden Seal, Myrrh and Lavender. Add two teaspoons of the combined mixture to 300 ml (½ pint) of boiling water, infuse for ten minutes then apply warm liquid to affected areas with a cotton wool swab.

| Aromatherapy Oils |

★ *Bath soak:* add two drops each of Sage, Lemon, Thyme and Tea Tree to a warm bath.

★ *Douche:* add one drop of Lavender oil to one litre (1¾ pints) of warm water and use as douche (do not do this too often).

TOOTHACHE

Tooth decay and abcesses are the two biggest causes of toothache. Decay is encouraged by bad dental hygiene and the wrong diet. Bacteria ferment sugary foods in the mouth into acids, these acids then eat away at the tooth enamel – this is when teeth have twinges. Eventually the pulp is exposed and the tooth dies. An abcess is extremely painful because it puts pressure on the tooth cavity by filling with pus. Usually the only way to remove an abcess is to take out the tooth or drain the pus.

Diet

To maintain optimum tooth health AVOID soft, sugary, refined foods that may stick to the teeth or leave an invisible layer of sugar on the enamel.

★ **DO NOT EAT**   sugary snacks in between meals.

★ **EAT**   lots of crunchy, raw vegetables which have an abrasive action on the teeth. Calcium is necessary for strong teeth so eat a moderate amount of cheese, milk, pulses, nuts and eggs.

Beneficial Supplements

For prevention of tooth decay:
Vitamin B6 (10 mg daily)
Vitamin A (up to 5000 IU daily)
Vitamin D (up to 400 IU daily)

Homoeopathy

Arnica 30c: after a filling, or injury to tooth
Silica 30c: pain from abcess
Belladonna 30c: throbbing pain in gums
Chamomilla 6c: very painful, sensitive to cold air

Herbal Remedies

★ *Direct application:*　chew raw Cloves.

Aromatherapy Oils

★ *Direct application:*　oil of Clove rubbed on to tooth.

TRAVEL SICKNESS

The motion of a boat, plane or car can all serve to make a susceptible person travel sick. The motion upsets the tiny balance system within the inner ear, which, in turn, causes nausea and vomiting. People who tend to suffer from travel sickness can also stimulate the feeling before they actually travel, because that is what they expect. Others suffer from phobias, flying for example, which bring on similar symptoms.

Diet

★ *AVOID*　spicy or fatty food prior to travelling.

★ *EAT A LITTLE*　plain food before travelling, it may help to settle the stomach, such as some wholemeal toast and butter or some fruit. Try taking some liver salts diluted in water before and during travel.

Beneficial Supplements

Raspberry leaf tablets

Homoeopathy

Chosen remedy to be taken every quarter of an hour, a couple of hours before travelling.

Tabacum 6c: nausea, sweating, shivering

Cocculus 6c: over–salivation, desire to lie down

Borax 6c: air travel
Nux Vomica 6c: queasy, headache, constipation, chilly

Herbal Remedies

★ *Infusion:*   (for tea) Ginger Root. In tablet, tincture or tea form, this is one of the best stomach calmers around. To make a tea, use one and a half teaspoons of ground ginger to a cupful of water, bring to boil and simmer for five minutes. With the fresh root, pour a mug of boiling water over one teaspoon of root and infuse for five minutes.

Aromatherapy Oils

★ *Inhalant:*   Peppermint oil freshens the air – sprinkle a couple of drops on to a hankie and place near mouth or nose.

VOMITING

The usual cause of vomiting is an irritant in the stomach, perhaps a bug, too much alcohol, or too much rich food. Vomiting can also be the result of emotional states such as revulsion.

For whatever reason, when the stomach receives the message to be sick from the brain, the muscles contract and send up semi-digested food. This can happen over and over again – for instance, in the case of food poisoning – until the irritant has been rejected.

Diet

★ *AVOID*   refined, rich, fatty and spicy foods, also tea and coffee which stimulate the gastric juices. When you vomit you can dehydrate quite easily, losing liquid, salt and minerals from the stomach.

★ **DRINK PLENTY** of liquids to replace those lost. If the vomiting is due to an infection, you will not be able to eat until the bug has been eliminated, and even then you will feel weak and have a small appetite.

★ **EAT** wholemeal bread with vegetable broth, protein foods such as a boiled egg, or piece of white fish. Live yogurt is very beneficial and should be eaten daily until better.

Beneficial Supplements

Vitamin C (1 g daily)
Vitamin B3 (also known as niacin, up to 100 mg daily)

Homoeopathy

Chosen remedy to be taken every half hour for up to ten doses per day.
Creosotum 6c: multiple attacks of vomiting
Nux Vomica 6c: after overeating or eating something you are allergic to
Arsenicum 6c: chilliness, diarrhoea – patient has to lie down
Ipecacuanha 6c: continuous feeling of nausea, pains in stomach

Herbal Remedies

★ **Infusion:** (for tea) Meadowsweet and Cinnamon. Add one teaspoon of Meadowsweet and a little Cinnamon to a cupful of boiling water, infuse for ten minutes, strain then drink. Or try Slippery Elm Food – made by adding one teaspoon of the powder to a beaten egg and adding a cupful of boiling milk to it. The drink can be flavoured with cinnamon or lemon rind.

Aromatherapy Oils

★ *Massage oil:*   add one drop of Lemon, one drop of Peppermint and one drop of Fennel to an eggcupful of Almond or Soya oil and massage into the upper abdomen.

WARTS AND VERRUCAE

Warts and verrucae belong to the same family of virus. They are small growths, usually round in shape, which can persist for some length of time, then suddenly disappear and heal of their own accord.

Verrucae, which occur on the soles of the feet, are known as 'plantar' warts and are dark brown in colour, whereas ordinary warts are red-looking or opaque.

The other kind of warts are relatively painless, but unsightly. Warts can be treated with freezing or corrosive substances, but the best action is just to let them heal of their own accord, and prevent them from returning.

Diet

★ *AVOID*   refined and processed foods.

★ *EAT PLENTY*   of foods containing Vitamin E and Vitamin A such as: Cod Liver oil, Olive oil, Halibut Liver oil, liver, fish, eggs, green leafy vegetables and pulses. Follow a basic wholefood diet, avoiding refined and processed foods.

Beneficial Supplements

Vitamin E (400 IU daily)
Anoint the skin with Vitamin E oil or lotion.

Homoeopathy

Tincture of Thuja: rub a little on to the wart, morning and evening

Herbal Remedies

★ *Skin application:* rub on juice from a Dandelion stem, apply Lemon juice or freshly crushed garlic. Do this twice a day.

Aromatherapy Oils

★ *Skin application:* rub a little oil of Lemon straight on to the wart or verruca.

REFERENCES

The Penguin Medical Encyclopaedia, Peter Wingate with Richard Wingate, third edition, Penguin, 1988.

Dictionary of Symptoms and Diseases, Richard B. Fisher, Corgi, 1988.

Alternative Medicine, Dr. Andrew Stanway, Penguin, 1986.

Thorsons Complete Guide to Vitamins and Minerals, Leonard Mervyn, Thorsons, 1986.

The Vitamin Bible, Earl Mindell, second edition, Arlington Books, 1985.

Health on Your Plate, Janet Pleshette, Hamlyn, 1983.

Nutritional Medicine, Dr. Stephen Davies and Dr Alan Stewart, Pan Books, 1987.

The Everyman Companion to Food and Nutrition, Sheila Bingham, Everyman, 1987.

The Dictionary of Vitamins, Leonard Mervyn, Thorsons, 1984.

Minerals: Their Crucial Role in Your Health, Miriam Polunin, Thorsons, 1987.

Herbal Medicine, Anne McIntyre, Macdonald Optima, 1987.

Mitton's Practical Herbal, F. & V. Mitton, Foulsham, 1976.

A Modern Herbal, Mrs M. Grieve, Penguin, 1931.

The Holistic Herbal, David Hoffmann, Findhorn, 1983.

Neal's Yard Natural Remedies, Susan Curtis, Romy Fraser, Irene Kohler, Arkana, 1988.

The Aromatherapy Handbook, Danièle Ryman, Century, 1984.

The Practice of Aromatherapy, Dr. Jean Valnet, C.W. Daniel, 1980.

Practical Aromatherapy, Shirley Price, Thorsons, 1983/87.

The Family Guide to Homoeopathy, Dr. Andrew Lockie, Elm Tree Books, 1989.

An Encyclopaedia of Homoeopathy, Dr. Trevor Smith, Insight Editions, 1983.

Homoeopathic Medicine, Dr. Trevor Smith, Thorsons, 1982.

Homoeopathy for Everyone, Drs. Sheila and Robin Gibson, Penguin Health.

Holistic First Aid, Dr. Michael Nightingale, Macdonald Optima, 1988.

FOOD FACTS

FAT

The main sources of fat are full cream milk, cheese, butter, margarine, fatty meats and fish, pastry, cakes and biscuits made with fat and fried foods. Although the greatest source of energy, fat intake should be limited as much as possible. Drink more skimmed milk, eat more lean meat and non-oily fish for better health.

PROTEIN

The main sources of protein are skimmed milk, yogurt, cheese, soya products, nuts, seeds, pulses, wholegrains, wheatgerm, sprouting seeds, meat, eggs and seafood. Protein is essential for a healthy immune system and helps to build muscle, cartilage, tendons, hair, nails and skin.

UNREFINED CARBOHYDRATES

The main sources of unrefined carbohydrates are potatoes, parsnips, wholemeal bread, wholewheat pasta, brown rice, bran, vegetables and dried fruit. Unrefined carbohydrate is a main source of energy and dietary fibre, which keeps the digestion and bowels working properly.

VITAMIN A

Essential for good sight, healthy skin and aids strong bone, teeth, hair and gum growth. Best food sources are halibut liver oil, liver, dairy products, eggs, yellow and orange fruit and vegetables.

VITAMIN B1 (Thiamine)

Helps digestion, ensures a healthy nervous system, muscles and heart. Best food sources are brewer's yeast, brown rice, wheatgerm, nuts and pork.

VITAMIN B2 (Riboflavin)

Repairs body tissues and mucous membranes, metabolises proteins, carbohydrates, fats, aids healthy skin, nails and hair. Best food sources are yeast extract, brewer's yeast, liver, cheese, green leafy vegetables and eggs.

VITAMIN B3 (Niacin)

Works towards healthy digestion, skin, nerves, brain and tongue. Best food sources are yeast extract, brewer's yeast, wheat bran, nuts, liver, white meat and fatty fish.

VITAMIN B5 (Pantothenic acid)

Combats fatigue, helps wounds heal, fights infection and produces anti-stress hormones. Best food sources are brewer's yeast, liver, nuts, wheat bran, wheat germ, soya flour, eggs and chicken.

VITAMIN B6 (Pyridoxine)

Promotes healthy skin and nerves, acts as an anti-depressant and may alleviate nausea. Best food sources are brewer's yeast, wheat bran, wheat germ, oatflakes, liver, soya flour, bananas and nuts.

VITAMIN B12 (Cobalamin)

Promotes energy, a healthy nervous system, and prevents anaemia. Best food sources are liver, kidney, fatty fish, pork, beef, eggs and cheese.

VITAMIN B (Complex)

This supplement contains all the B vitamins, plus a number of other complementary substances such as choline, inositol, folic acid and biotin.

VITAMIN C

Increases resistance to infection, produces anti-stress hormones, decreases blood cholesterol, helps in the absorption of iron, and up-keep of collagen. Best food sources are cherry juice, rosehip syrup, black-currants, citrus fruits and green leafy vegetables.

VITAMIN D

Essential for strong bones and teeth and helps prevent colds. Best food sources are cod liver oil, herring, mackerel, sardines, tuna, canned salmon, eggs and milk.

VITAMIN E

Antioxidant which promotes healthy blood vessels, supplies oxygen, prevents blood clots, and when directly applied to skin has a healing effect. Best food sources are wheatgerm oil, soya bean oil and vegetable oils.

INDEX